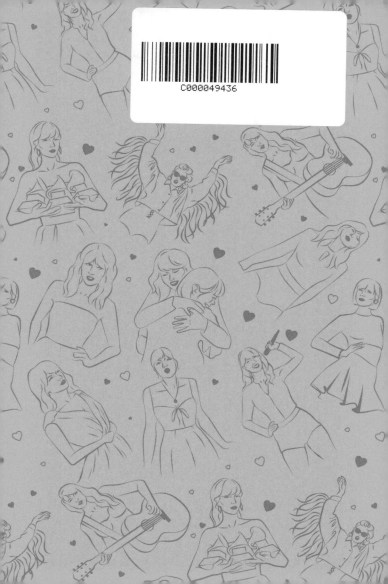

- LINES TO LIVE BY -

TAYLOR SWIFT

Shake it off and love yourself with Taylor's
best inspirational quotes

POP PRESS

Published in 2022 by Pop Press, an imprint of Ebury Publishing,
20 Vauxhall Bridge Road,
London SW1V 2SA

Pop Press is part of the Penguin Random House group of companies
whose addresses can be found at global.penguinrandomhouse.com

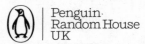

www.penguin.co.uk

A CIP catalogue record for this book is available from the British Library

Design: Seagull Design
Text: Charlotte Cole
Illustrations: LJG Designs

ISBN 9781529149395

Printed and bound in Great Britain by Clays Ltd, Elcograf S.p.A.

The authorised representative in the EEA is Penguin Random House Ireland,
Morrison Chambers, 32 Nassau Street, Dublin D02 YH68

CONTENTS

TAYLOR'S LINES TO LIVE BY

Swifties know that Taylor kills it.

Getting her first job as a songwriter aged 13, Taylor Swift's rise to being one of the bestselling music artists of all time has been nothing short of meteoric. She's a non-stop creative mastermind and an outstanding businesswoman. She's also never short of an epic clap back when she needs to stand up for what's right.

This book is crammed with wisdom from the woman herself. If you need a helping hand or a confidence boost, or you are worrying about love or the friends in your life, Taylor's words will speak to you. With her views on creativity and hard work, and how to handle success when it arrives, it has everything you need for an empowered and inspired life.

You are never, ever getting better advice than you'll find in these pages, so shake off the bad times and take on the world the Tay Tay way.

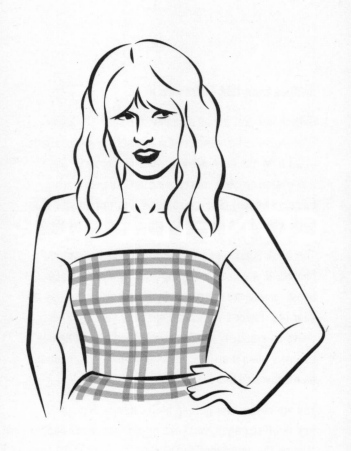

CONFIDENCE

'Lately I've been focusing less on doing what they say I can't do and more on doing whatever the hell I want.'

'My definition of "fearless" is not that you're not afraid. It's that you're afraid but you jump anyway.'

'Anytime you're standing up against or for anything, you're never going to receive unanimous praise. But that's what forces you to be brave.'

'If you think too hard about who other people want you to be as an artist, it stops you from being who you want to be as an artist.'

'Growing up and knowing that I was an adult was realising that I was allowed to take up space from a marketing perspective, from a business perspective, from an opinionated perspective.'

'That's kind of the nature of a live performance. You know, things could go wrong. That's part of the excitement of being there.'

'I try really hard to keep it light. Joy, enthusiasm, excitement – those are sort of my chief attributes.'

'I don't think you should ever have to apologise for your excitement. Just because something's clichéd doesn't mean that it's not something that's awesome.'

'There might be times when you put your whole heart and soul into something and it is met with cynicism or scepticism – you cannot let that crush you. [. . .] Please remember that you have the right to prove them wrong.'

'The only real risk is being
too afraid to take a risk
at all.'

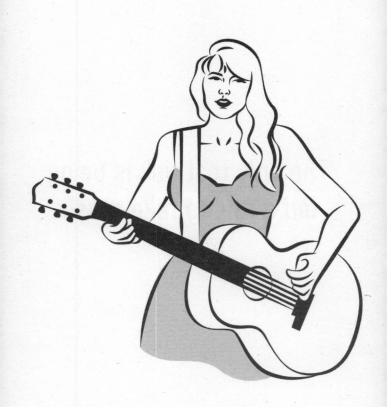

CREATIVITY

'There are definitely moments when it's like this cloud of an idea comes and just lands in front of your face, and you reach up and grab it.'

'For me, it starts as an idea and a feeling or an emotion.'

'It's all trying to figure out how to say things in a way I've never said them, how to make them sound the way I've never made them sound before.'

'I think as a songwriter there is this urge to connect. There is that urge to say this is how I feel sometimes, and then have fans say, "Oh my god, I feel that way sometimes too." '

'I grew up just understanding metaphor and just kind of loving how you could take something you're going through and speak about it in a different way that applies how you're feeling to something completely different.'

'Samples and beat-dropping and pointless collaborations [. . .] there are a lot of different ways that you can get distracted from the fact that people just want to listen to a good song.'

'Write your songs not for a specific demographic or for getting on the radio or for anything commercial like that. Write your songs to the person you're writing that song about.'

'That's how I designed these clues, so that different ones would reveal themselves over time. I know this makes me sound like a frustrating, magical elf making people guess my name or something.'

'Being a songwriter means
you're very attuned
to your own intuition and
your own feelings even
if they hurt.'

'It's so imperative for me as a human being that songwriting is not tied to my own personal misery. It's good to know that, it really is!'

'As an artist you try to change, just to evolve, for the sake of keeping things exciting for your fans, keeping things exciting for you.'

'That's the wonderful thing about trying as many different ways of writing music as possible; discoveries.'

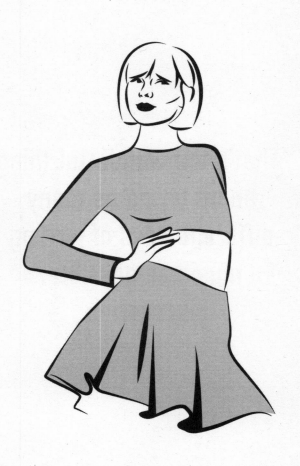

WORK IT

'Creativity is getting inspiration and having that lightning-bolt idea moment, and then having the hard work ethic to sit down at the desk and write it down.'

'You can be accidentally successful for three or four years. Accidents happen. But careers take hard work.'

'From the time I was about 9 years old I was doing theatre productions every time I got a chance, I was performing in cafes and writing songs and recording demos [. . .] Looking back I feel a bit weird about it as it doesn't feel normal for a kid, but it felt normal to me.'

'The reason I was so driven was that I didn't expect that anything would just happen for me. But that doubt fuelled me to work harder.'

'My parents raised me to have the mentality that you're not going to get anything unless you work for it [. . .] so I've just always worked really hard, played a lot of shows, tried to get out in front of as many people as possible.'

'I signed my publishing deal at age 14 [. . .] I knew that I had to work just as hard as the veteran 45-year-old writers who were also signed there.'

'You become a brand as soon as you sell one thing, so you can either recognise it and embrace it or you can deny it and pretend it's not happening.'

'What I've always wanted to do, and my main goal above everything else, is to beat what I've done before. To me that's the most important thing.'

'I'll take a red-eye and do an interview, then go to a meet-and-greet, then do an appearance, then get ready for a show, then do a conference call about the album . . . My brain does get fried, but I never get tired of this.'

'[I'm] always putting forth this constant obstacle course for myself because it's exciting for me.'

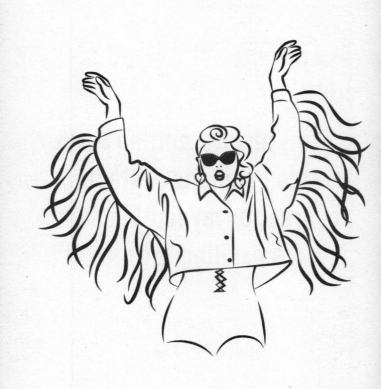

EQUALITY

'[Women in music] are held to a higher, sometimes impossible-feeling standard. And it feels like my fellow female artists have taken this challenge and they have accepted it. It seems that the pressure that could have crushed us made us into diamonds instead.'

'I think it happens to women so often that, as we get older and see how the world works, we're able to see through what is gaslighting.'

'If a guy shares his experience in writing, he's brave. If a woman shares her experience in writing, she's oversharing. And she's over-emotional, or she might be crazy [. . .] that joke is so old, and it's coming from a place of such sexism.'

'There's a different vocabulary for men and women [. . .] A man does something, it's strategic. A woman does the same thing, it's calculated. A man is allowed to react, a woman can only overreact.'

'You should not be blamed for waiting 15 minutes or 15 days or 15 years to report sexual assault or harassment, or for the outcome of what happens to a person after he or she makes the choice to sexually harass or assault you.'

'What we need in any fight for equality, in any group of people, is we need people from the other side to say, "Yeah, you're right. You're right to want that."'

'I love showing that we really do have allies in the male civilisation.'

'My hope for the future, not just in the music industry, but in every young girl I meet . . . is that they all realise their worth and ask for it.'

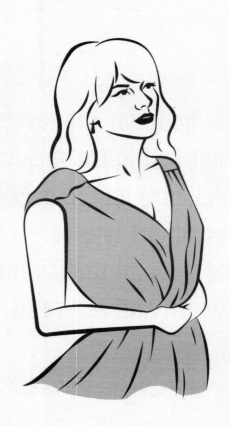

MENTAL
HEALTH

'You can be vulnerable
and lonely and
independent and strong
and brave and scared all
at once.'

'You can't micromanage
life, it turns out.'

'Our priorities can get messed up existing in a society that puts a currency on curating the way people see your life.'

'My relationship with food was exactly the same psychology that I applied to everything else in my life: If I was given a pat on the head, I registered that as good. If I was given a punishment, I registered that as bad.'

'I'm a woman, I'm not a coathanger. I need to feel healthy in my life, I need to take pleasure in food, and I need to not use my body as an exercise in control when I feel out of control in my life.'

'I think social dynamics of walking into a cafeteria and not knowing where to sit is kind of like an important human experience.'

'I've never ever felt edgy, cool or sexy. Not one time. [. . .] It's not important for [teenage girls] to be those things. It's important for them to be imaginative, intelligent, hardworking, strong, smart, quick-witted, charming.'

'I realised I needed to restructure my life because it felt completely out of control . . . I knew immediately I needed to make music about it because I knew it was the only way I could survive it.'

'I try to encourage my fans that they don't have to feel confident every day, they don't have to feel happy every day [. . .] They shouldn't put added, extra pressure on themselves to feel happy when they're not, you know?'

'We are heartbroken the same way and we fall in love the same way and we are happy the same way and the fact that you would listen to my music means that we're on the same page.'

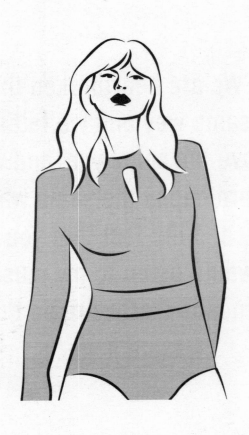

RESILIENCE

'Do I feel more balanced in my life than I ever have before? Um, probably, yeah. But is that permanent? No. And I think being okay with that has put me in a bit of a better position.'

'I still am someone who is the first to apologise when I'm wrong, but I think I'm better at standing up for myself when I've been wronged.'

'If you make the joke first and you make the joke better, then it's not as funny when other people call you a name.'

'There was this crazy circumstance that happened where I wrote this song "Mean" about the harshest criticisms I've ever gotten. It was brutal. And that song ended up winning two Grammys.'

'It's my way of coping . . .
I write when I'm
frustrated, angry or
confused. I've figured out
a way to filter all of that
into something good.'

'The thing about being a songwriter is that no matter what happens, if you write a song about it, it's productive.'

'I think that you learn a lot of lessons as you're growing up, and one of them has to be human compassion.'

'As long as you're having more fun than anyone else, what does it matter what anyone else thinks?'

'The bad stuff was really significant and damaging. But the good stuff will endure.'

'I can live my life without any public approval and still have a really really wonderful life.'

'You have to understand and appreciate something cool when it happens to you. It's like, little victories you have to celebrate.'

'As soon as you fail, enthusiasm tells you that the next great idea is around the corner.'

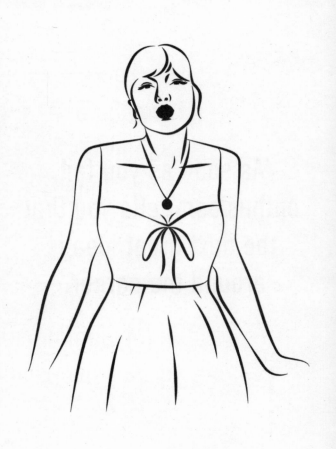

LOVE

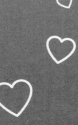

'Today you're heartbroken,
but tomorrow you'll be in
love again.'

'When we're falling in love or out of it, that's when we most need a song that says how we feel. Yeah, I write a lot of songs about boys. And I'm very happy to do that.'

'This album [*Lover*] is really a love letter to love, in all of its maddening, passionate, exciting, enchanting, horrific, tragic, wonderful glory.'

'If you think too hard
about it and it takes you a
long time to fall in love
with someone you're not
in *love* love.'

'I have a lot of rules placed on my life and I just choose not to apply rules to love.'

'You know when people say "I saw him and I just KNEW" when they meet the one? Yeah, I walk around saying that about a cat.'

'I think it's healthy for everyone to go a few years without dating, just because you need to get to know who you are.'

'They have to be a good guy [. . .] That's the new thing I'm working on.'

'The way I look at love is that it's all going to be bad until it's good, you know?'

'I just love talking about love. I love writing about love. I love thinking about love because it's so unpredictable.'

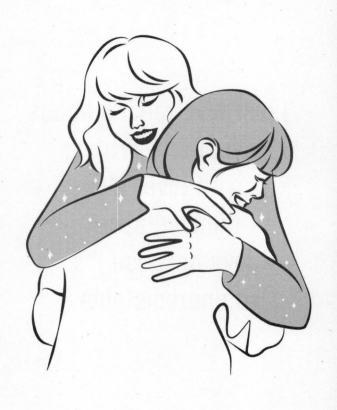

FRIENDS

'I now see resilience as a major quality in friendship. Like when your stock is down, if they're still wanting to hang out, that's like 👌'

'It makes it less like work, having your friends out there [on tour].'

'It was important to show that losing friendships can be just as damaging to a person as losing a romantic relationship.'

'One thing you have to do
as a friend is be there for
them no matter what
they're going through
and never try to boss
them around.'

'I'm pleasantly surprised by the fact that I tell my friends absolutely everything and it never ends up getting out.'

'Some of my best friendships came from people publicly criticising me and then it opening up a conversation.'

'One thing about learning to be the best friend you can possibly be is knowing when you have to let people figure things out on their own.'

'I surround myself with smart, beautiful, passionate, driven, ambitious women. Other women who are killing it should motivate you, thrill you, challenge you and inspire you.'

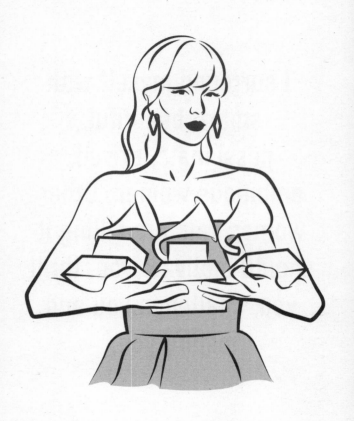

WOMEN
WHO
INSPIRE

'Becoming friends with Lena [Dunham] . . . just seeing why she believes what she believes, why she says what she says, why she stands for what she stands for – has made me realise that I've been taking a feminist stance without actually saying so.'

'What Annie [Lennox] does is so interesting to me, and it's not something you could ever try to duplicate. But the way she conveys a thought, there's something really intense about it. And I think that's something I'll always aspire to.'

'Over the course of her career [Diana Ross] has stood up for herself so many times, in a time when it was not popular for a woman to stand up for herself.'

'The Dixie Chicks were always having so much fun, and writing their own songs, and playing their own instruments, and I think that's what I wanted to follow.'

'I love people like Jameela Jamil, because the way she speaks about body image, it's almost like she speaks in a hook [. . .] it gets stuck in my head and it calms me down.'

'Halsey's an amazing writer, and she speaks up for what she cares about and she's very vocal about things [. . .] We have these very fierce women out there.'

The way that [Lana Wilson] so artfully manoeuvred through such a touchy subject [in *After Tiller*], with such emotional intelligence, that's what made me such a fan.

'Shania Twain is just *so* independent and confident and empowering.'

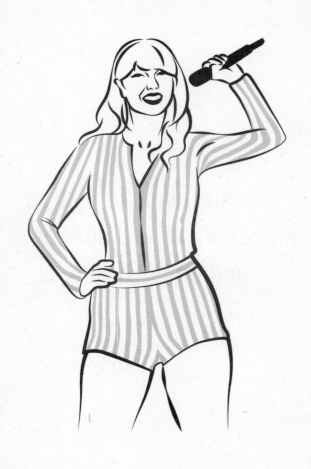

SUCCESS

'I really try to live in the moment and be really stoked about everything that happens, but never feel entitled for it to keep happening. So when it does keep happening I'm just really excited about it.'

'My life is never the same two days in a row. It's never routine [. . .] This job was perfect for me because I love that adventure!'

'The cool thing about my job is that it's very spontaneous. You have to get used to not getting used to things.'

'All we have are our memories, and our hope for future memories [. . .] I just like to hopefully give people a soundtrack to those things.'

'[This AMA Artist of the Year Award] represents encouragement and motivation for me to be better, work harder and try to make you guys proud as much as I possibly can.'

'I've never felt entitled to ever get to play another sold-out show or get nominated for another award or win another award or – you know, right now is all you're really guaranteed to have.'

'I have definitely made decisions that have made my life feel more like a real life and less like just a storyline to be commented on in tabloids. [. . .] it's really just trying to find bits of normalcy.'

'You have to look around you every day, and take note of the people who have always believed in you and never stop appreciating them for it. Never take them for granted.'

'When I hear the crowd screaming I just get so happy. It's like the most amazing sound. I just stand there and take it in sometimes, because it's in those moments that I realise that's part of the highlight reel for when I'm like 80 years old.'

On fans:
'It's me and it's them, and that's what makes it fun for me.'

'There are two things that have protected me over the course of my career. And the first thing is enthusiasm. And the second is how much I love music.'

'Now I get to choose when I work, I get to choose the things I wanna work on, and I don't take that for granted – ever.'

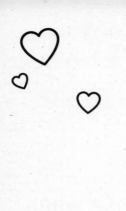

ACKNOWLEDGEMENTS

P2 from acceptance speech, Billboard Woman of the Decade Award (2019), P3 from City Life, Phillymag.com, 'Exit interview: Taylor Swift' (2008), P4 from *Variety*, 'No Longer "Polite At All Costs"' (2020), P5 from the *Wall Street Journal*, 'Is Taylor Swift Still a Country Artist? Let's Ask Taylor Swift' (2012), P6 from *Music Week*, 'I come with opinions about how we can better our industry' (2019), P7 from *All Access Nashville with Katie Couric* (2013), P8 from *Esquire*, 'Why Taylor Swift Welcomed You to New York' (2014), P9 from BBC Radio 1 Live Lounge interview (2019), P10 from acceptance speech, BRITs Global Icon Award (2021), P11 from the *Wall Street Journal*, 'For Taylor Swift, the Future of Music Is a Love Story' (2014), P14 from *Harper's BAZAAR*, 'Taylor Swift Interviews Rock 'n' Roll Icon Pattie Boyd on Songwriting, Beatlemania, & the Power of Being a Muse' (2018), P15 From *YouTube Presents Taylor Swift* (2011), P16 from CMT, *Hot 20 Countdown* (2012), P17 from Netflix Film Club, *Taylor Swift Breaks Down her Creative Process: Miss Americana* (2020), P18 from *YouTube Presents Taylor Swift* (2011), P19 from *Wonderland*, 'Taylor' Swift' (2014), P20 from *TIME Magazine Interviews: Taylor Swift* (2009), P21 from *Independent*, 'What you didn't know about ME!' (2019), P22 from *Time*, 'Taylor Swift on *1989*, Spotify, Her Next Tour and Female Role Models' (2014), P23 from *Music Week*, 'I come with opinions about how we can better our industry' (2019), P24 from *Today Show* Australia interview (2012), P25 from *Wonderland.*, 'Taylor' Swift' (2014), P28 from *Vogue*, '73 Questions With Taylor Swift' (2016), P29 from *GQ*, 'Taylor Swift on "Bad Blood," Kanye West, and How People Interpret Her Lyrics (2015), P30 from *SABC Top Billing* (2014), P31 from Seventeen.com, 'Five Questions with Taylor Swift' (2009), P32 from *The Hot Desk* (2014), P33 from *SongwriterUniverse*, 'Taylor Swift Discusses Her Debut Album, Early Hits, And How She Got Started' (2007), P34 from *All Access Nashville with Katie Couric* (2013), P35 from iTunes interview, *Taylor Swift – Fearless Platinum Edition* (2009), P36 from *Women's Health*, 'She's Living Her Taylor-Made Dream' (2008), P37 from BBC Radio 1 *Live Lounge* interview (2019), P40 from acceptance speech, Billboard Woman of the Decade Award (2019), P41 from *Guardian*, 'I was literally about to break' (2019), P42 from ABC News, *Barbra Walters Most Fascinating People* (2014), P43 from CBS News, 'Taylor Swift on "Lover" and haters' (2019), P44 from *Time*, '"I Was Angry." Taylor Swift on What Powered Her Sexual Assault Testimony' (2017), P45 from *On Air With Ryan Seacrest*, 'Taylor Swift Talks Newfound "Freedom," "Lover" Tour Plans and So Much More' (2019), P46 from Netflix Film Club, *Taylor Swift Breaks Down her Creative Process: Miss Americana* (2020), P47 from the *Wall Street Journal*, 'For Taylor Swift, the Future of Music Is a Love Story' (2014), P50 from *WSJ Magazine*, 'The Ballad of Selena Gomez' (2020), P51 from *Guardian*, 'I was literally about to break' (2019), P52 from *Entertainment Weekly*, 'Taylor Swift shares intel on TS7, fan theories, and her next era' (2019), P53 from Variety.com, 'Taylor Swift Opens Up About Overcoming Struggle With Eating Disorder' (2020), P54 from British *Vogue*, 'Taylor Swift Tries Out Her Best British Slang On Edward Enninful' (2019), P55 from *The Bobby Bones Show* (2013), P56 from NPR, '"Anything That Connects": A Conversation With Taylor Swift' (2014), P57 from *Vogue*, 'Taylor Swift on Sexism, Scrutiny, and Standing Up for Herself' (2019), P58 from *Genius*, '1989 Interview with Paul McGuire' (2014), P59 from acceptance speech AMA Artist of the Year Award (2013), P62 from *Entertainment Weekly*, 'Taylor Swift shares intel on TS7, fan theories, and her next era' (2019), P63 from CBS News, 'Taylor Swift on "Lover" and haters' (2019), P64 from Global News, *Taylor Swift: Reacts to being named the voice of her generation* (2014), P65 from *Genius*, '1989 Interview with Paul McGuire' (2014), P66 from *Women's Health*, 'She's Living Her Taylor-Made Dream' (2008), P67 from City Life, Phillymag.com, 'Exit interview: Taylor Swift' (2008), P68 from *The New Yorker*, 'You Belong with Me' (2011), P69 from *Guardian*, 'Taylor Swift: "Sexy? Not on my radar"' (2014), P70 from *Rolling Stone*, 'The Rolling Stone Interview Taylor Swift' (2019), P71 from BBC Radio 1 Live Lounge interview (2019), P72 from BBC Radio 1 *Live Lounge* interview (2014), P73 from *Entertainment Weekly*, 'Taylor Swift Blown Away by Support of Fans as She Accepts Gracie Award for 'Folklore' Concert Film' (2021), P76 from Seventeen.com, 'Five Questions with Taylor Swift' (2009), P77 from *Guardian*, 'Taylor Swift: 'I want to believe in pretty lies' (2012), P78 from *Vogue*, 'Taylor Swift on Sexism, Scrutiny, and Standing Up for Herself' (2019), P79 from *The Jonathan Ross Show* (2012), P80 from *The Jonathan Ross Show* (2012), P81 from *Independent*, 'What you didn't know about ME!' (2019), P82 from *Esquire*, 'Why Taylor Swift Welcomed You to New York' (2014), P83 from *Taylor Swift Interview Backstage at the Capital FM Summertime Ball* (2013), P84 from *The Times*, 'Don't mess with Taylor Swift' (2013), P85 from *Country Weekly*, 'Taylor Swift Talks Writing, Relationships, Rejects and New Album "Red"' (2012), P88 from Apple Music, *Taylor Swift: 'Lover' and Attending an Emo Dinner Party* (2019), P89 from *Taylor Swift Interview Backstage at the Capital FM Summertime Ball* (2013), P90 from *GQ*, 'Taylor Swift on "Bad Blood," Kanye West, and How People Interpret Her Lyrics (2015), P91 from 2DayFMSydney, Jules, Merrick & Sophie (2014), P92 from *Vogue*, '73 Questions With Taylor Swift' (2016), P93 from *Rolling Stone*, 'The *Rolling Stone* Interview Taylor Swift' (2019), P94 From 2DayFMSydney, Jules, Merrick & Sophie (2014), P95 from *Time*, 'Taylor Swift on 1989, Spotify, Her Next Tour and Female Role Models' (2014), P98 from *Guardian*, 'Taylor Swift: "Sexy? Not on my radar"' (2014), P99 from NPR, '"Anything That Connects": A Conversation With Taylor Swift' (2014), P100 from acceptance speech for AMA Dick Clark Award for Excellence (2014), P101 from *Today Show* Australia interview (2012), P102 from *Variety*, 'No Longer "Polite At All Costs"' (2020), P103 from Apple Music, *Taylor Swift: 'Lover' and Attending an Emo Dinner Party* (2019), P104 from *Taylor Swift: Miss Americana – Sundance 2020 World Premiere Q&A* (2002), P105 from iTunes interview, *Taylor Swift – Fearless Platinum Edition* (2009), P108 from CityTV Canada interview (2019), P109 from *Country Weekly*, 'Taylor Swift Talks Writing, Relationships, Rejects and New Album "Red"' (2012), P110 from ITV, *Lorraine* (2014), P111 from *Guardian*, 'Taylor Swift: "I want to believe in pretty lies" (2012), P112 from acceptance speech AMA Artist of the Year Award (2018), P113 from Billboard's Woman of the Year interview (2011), P114 from *Rolling Stone*, 'Paul McCartney & Taylor Swift' (2020), P115 from acceptance speech, BRITs Global Icon Award (2021), P116 from CityTV Canada interview (2019), P117 from Apple Music, *Taylor Swift: 'ME!' Interview* (2019), P118 from *Entertainment Weekly*, 'Taylor Swift Blown Away by Support of Fans as She Accepts Gracie Award for 'Folklore' Concert Film' (2021), P119 from British *Vogue*, 'Taylor Swift Tries Out Her Best British Slang On Edward Enninful' (2019)

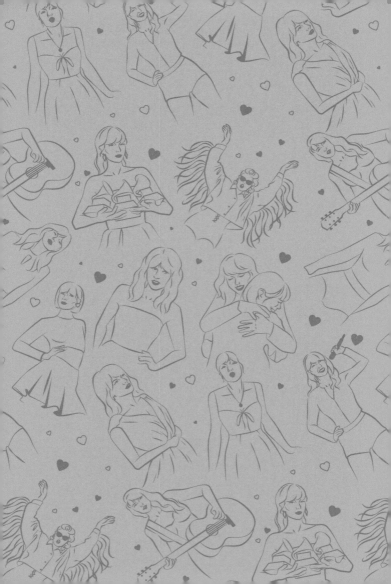